I0789842

INTERMITTENT FASTING:

A GUIDE FOR LOSING WEIGHT, RESETTING YOUR METABOLISM AND STAYING HEALTHY FOR LIFE

Eden Fancher

TABLE OF CONTENTS

INTRODUCTION TO INTERMITTENT FASTING

Intermittent fasting involves alternating periods of feast and famine in which you may eat as much as you like during the feasting, but drink only water or other non-nutritive drinks during the fast. The aim is to achieve the benefits of calorie reduction and for some, use it as vehicle to lose weight.

Intermittent fasting can be done in a number of ways, in alternating 24 hour periods or daily. The first option requires that you abstain from some or all meals on one or more days of the week. Daily fasting utilizes 24 hour periods of eating and fasting that begin and end at the same time each day; for example, fast from Monday 6pm until Tuesday 6pm, eat as much as you like from Tuesday 6pm to Wednesday 6pm and repeat the process. During daily intermittent fasting, there is a short period for eating, usually 4-6 hours within the 24 hour day, during which you can eat as much as you like.

Some of the things that put people off are the fear that they will be extremely hungry and not stick to the plan, or do not know how to fit it into their schedule. This is actually quite simple; if you plan in advance, you get to eat your evening meal at pretty much the same time every day, but at an hour either side, depending if you're on an intermittent fasting phase, or an eating phase. Again with a little planning, you can also accommodate socializing and eating out.

The main factor preventing many people from trying is the fear of being hungry. Although, this does take a little will power and a slight degree of discomfort to begin with, it will actually get easy!

WHAT IS FASTING?

Fasting is a willing abstinence or reduction from some or all food, drink, or both, for a period of time. An absolute fast (dry fasting) is normally defined as abstinence from all food and liquid for a defined period, usually a period of 24 hours, or a number of days. Water fasting allows drinking water, but nothing else. Other fasts may be partially restrictive, limiting only some particular foods or substances. A fast may also be intermittent in nature. Fasting practices may preclude intercourse and other activities, as well as food.

In a physiological context, fasting may refer to the metabolic status of a person who has not eaten overnight, or to the metabolic state achieved after complete digestion and absorption of a meal. Several metabolic adjustments occur during fasting, and some diagnostic tests are used to determine a fasting state. For example, a person is assumed to be fasting after 8–12 hours from their last meal. Metabolic changes toward the fasting state begin after absorption of a meal (typically 3–5 hours after a meal); "post-absorptive state" is synonymous with this usage, in contrast to the postprandial state of ongoing digestion.

A diagnostic fast refers to prolonged fasting (from 8–72 hours depending on age) conducted under observation for investigation of a problem, usually hypoglycemia.
Many people may also fast as part of a medical procedure or check-up, such as a colonoscopy.

Fasting is also a part of many religious rituals.

Medical application of IF

Fasting is often practiced prior to surgery or other procedures that require general anesthetics, because of the risk of pulmonary aspiration of gastric contents after induction of anesthesia (i.e., vomiting and inhaling the vomit, causing life-threatening aspiration pneumonia). Additionally, certain medical tests, such as cholesterol testing (lipid panel) or certain blood glucose measurements, require fasting for several hours so that a baseline can be established. In the case of a lipid panel, failure to fast for a full 12 hours (including vitamins) will guarantee an elevated triglyceride measurement.

Cancer

Fasting is of no help in either preventing or treating cancer.
The American Cancer Society recommends that people undergoing chemotherapy should increase their intake of protein and calories; current research around dietary restriction in these circumstances are inconclusive – there is weak evidence that a short-term period of fasting may have benefits during treatment.

Mental health

Fasting can help alleviate some symptoms of depression. However, the psychological effects may also include anxiety and depression.

Immune system

Some scientists have indicated that a fast will cause white blood cells to break down during the fasting, resulting in new ones needing to be built when the fast is broken, resulting in the replacement of old damaged ones.

Weight loss

Although fasting will lead to weight loss, using fasting for weight loss is considered unnecessary.

Variations of fasting

Fasting is the act of willingly abstaining from food and sometimes, drink for a duration of time. A typical fast is just abstaining from food. Fluids are consumed in ample quantity to satisfy thirst and physiological requirements.
There are several different variations of fasting. These include:

Water Fasting/Juice Fasting/Fruit Fasting

The purpose of fasting (other than religious reasons) is a systematic cleansing of the body. During a fast, the body will cleanse itself of everything except vital tissues. The depth of the cleansing depends on the type and duration of fast.

Glucose is the body's primary source of fuel, and it's essential for brain functioning. When glucose is denied for over 4-8 hours, the body uses glycogen stored in the liver. Small amounts of protein are used to supplement the glycogen. This fuel source will last up to 12 hours.

Next, the body will use glycogen stored in the muscles; lasting a few more days. If glucose is still lacking at this point, the body switches to use fat as its primary fuel source (this prevents any muscle wasting). Fat is converted into ketones; ketones are not sugar but they can be used by the brain as a fuel source when glucose is not present.

It is important to note that starvation will NOT occur until the body is forced to use vital tissue to survive. A healthy person fasting for 40 days on just water will not suffer a deficiency of vitamins, minerals, proteins or fatty acids. The breakdown of unhealthy cells provides all the essential substances. The number of muscle fibers will remain constant. Healthy cells may be reduced in size and strength for a time; ultimately, they remain perfectly functional.

Human fat is valued at 3,500 calories per pound. Each pound of fat will supply more than enough energy for one day of hard physical labor. A study at the University of Chicago, states that a healthy, well-nourished man can live from 50 to 75 days without food. Provided he is not exposed to harsh elements or emotional stress.

The vast majority of people that fast discover that when they are fasting, they have no hunger and more energy. The reason behind this is detoxification. Detoxification is a normal body procedure that is enhanced during a fast. It's the eliminating or neutralizing of toxins through the colon, liver, kidneys, lungs, lymph glands and skin.

The first few days of a fast are the hardest. The first stage of detoxing removes large quantities of digestive residues and waste matter. The quantity of waste passing into the blood stream results in the tongue becoming coated and breath unpleasant, as the body excretes waste wherever it can. After the third day of the fast, hunger passes; there is little craving for food. The second stage of the fasting is cleansing of mucus, fat, disease, dead and dying cells, and lastly, toxins that have been accumulating in cellular tissue.

An extended fast removes: unwanted fatty tissue, trans-fatty acids, hardened coating of mucus on the intestinal wall; toxic waste matter in the blood stream, and lymphatic system; toxins in the spleen, liver and kidney; mucus from the lungs and sinuses; toxins embedded in the cellular fibers, and deeper organ tissues.

Fasting - How to Set Up a Daily Fasting Diet

Daily fasting is becoming more and more popular as a fat loss method, because of the quick results it provides and also because it is both easy to set up and, more importantly, easy to stick to long term. In fact, daily fasting can be both a short-term solution, and a long-term lifestyle for permanent physique changes and good health.

So how can you incorporate daily fasting? The first thing to do is to decide how long it should be. Most effective plans range from 16-24 hours, followed by a "re-feeding period" that can be anywhere from 8-24 hours. This decision can adapt to you, rather than forcing you to make big lifestyle changes in order to fit in with the demands of an eating plan, something that is common in most diets.

After establishing the length of the daily fasting period depending on goals and lifestyle, the start and end points of the fast need to be decided. This is where the ease intermittent fasting becomes apparent. For example, with an eight hour feeding "window", a good plan might be to eat from 12.30 to 8.30 in the evening, and then fast until the next day at 12.30 (lunchtime). Why is this an easy system to put into practice? Simply because, it is not that different to what most people do anyway. Eat an evening meal, skip breakfast and then, start eating again at lunch the next day.

The other question to ask yourself about daily fasting would be food choices. Again, here is another big advantage. Most other fat loss plans you care to mention will basically rule out a huge number of things that you want to eat. This is not a good idea for all sorts of reasons, particularly the effect this has on leptin, a crucial hormone in fat loss.

This diet is far less severe in terms of food choice. Whilst re-feeding on soda and burgers is not a good idea, certain foods that wouldn't normally be associated with fat loss are fine here and in fact, will even help your diet.

WHAT IS INTERMITTENT FASTING?

"Intermittent fasting" is a term used to describe ways you can manipulate your eating patterns. It involves not eating for specific periods of time, with the intent to lose weight and improve health. Intermittent fasting can include anything from multiday fast to skipping meals a few times a week. Many people consider it appealing because it doesn't involve large daily calorie restriction.

Fasting is a practice that is centuries old, spanning across cultures, religions and countries. There have been claims that intermittent fasting offers other health benefits besides weight loss, such as:

- Improving the body's sensitivity to insulin

- Lowering inflammation

- Improving the digestive system

- Reducing body fat

While some research does show short-term benefits such as these, more studies are needed to confirm these findings. Much remains to be learned about the long-term health effects of intermittent fasting.

In one study, fasting helped halt the spread of intestinal bacteria into the bloodstream. Researchers have also suggested that the positive results from fasting can help with brain function.

What Is Intermittent Fasting, and How Can You to Apply It to Your Life

Losing weight is something that a lot of people all over the world are facing the problems of. But what most people fail to realize is that intermittent fasting is the best approach that you can use to really help you lose weight when you are struggling to get those pounds lost. Losing weight is, and should not, be hard. People make a big deal out of something that should be a slow and enjoyable process that everyone can enjoy.

Intermittent fasting and fasting in general, is known throughout the world as something that is very good for the health. But people in general, do not want to go anywhere near it. People find that fasting is something that people will struggle with, but the great thing about intermittent fasting is that you only do it on occasion. Plus, in a day, doing fasting every once in a while is a great way to get past that plateau that you may have hit with losing the excess weight that you have on you.

The best way that you can apply intermittent fasting to your life is to start slowly, and gradually increase the time that you do it. This way, you will allow your body to get used to the whole process, and you will see the results without having to overwhelm yourself. So the key is to start slow, and slowly increase the amount of time that you do it. Make sure that you do not do it more than once a week for maximum benefits.

Another thing that you need to take into consideration is that intermittent fasting is not the only thing that you are going to have to do to effectively lose weight. This has to be part of a big program that you are going to use in order to live a more healthy life. You need to make sure that your diet is perfect, and you need to make sure that you are implementing a proper exercise routine into your life. Only when these things are perfect that you're are going to find out that you will be seeing the long term results that you are after. Intermittent fasting is not an end to itself, but something that must be a part of a bigger strategy. This is the only way you are going to be successful.

How to Start

Seeking the help of a professional is advisable before you start fasting. However, you can start by choosing a day to skip breakfast. You can choose to have water, black coffee or tea in lieu of breakfast. As you progress, try to go further by skipping lunch. If you feel that you need to eat or are feeling anxious, you can take a normal sized meal.

Keep in mind that intermittent fasting means that you take a break from eating so that your body will be able to produce hormones which can have a better effect on your cells for a better and longer life.

Things You Probably Don't Know About Intermittent Fasting

1. Intermittent Fasting (also referred to as I.F.), though given a pretty cool and somewhat exotic name, is simply the term that nutrition experts give to going certain extended periods of time without eating.

2. We all practice a form of intermittent fasting practically every day...when we sleep! That's right. From your last meal of the evening until your first meal the next day, you are practicing a form of intermittent fasting.

3. Though there is still lots of research left to do on intermittent fasting, some potential benefits include reduced blood pressure, reduced risk of some cancers, increased metabolic rate (think increased fat burning potential), and improved blood sugar control and cardiovascular functioning.

4. There are many different styles of I.F. programs. Some include one or more full fasting days (that's at least 24 hours straight without food) while some follow a less dramatic approach, such as the Leangains approach (16-hour fast/8-hour feed).

5. Intermittent fasting is not for the faint of heart. Before considering I.F., you should first understand the basic fundamentals for healthy weight loss and good nutrition. That being said, if you are a more advanced dieter and exerciser looking for a new and challenging way to burn fat, I.F. might be worth checking out. Just be aware that it will take sound planning and discipline to follow some of these approaches.

BENEFITS OF INTERMITTENT FASTING

Intermittent Fasting or IF for short is not a diet or starvation process. It is an eating pattern. When one fasts and also reduces their calorie intake, it can lead to a healthier and prolonged life. Take note that our ancestors before us were gatherers and hunters. They did not have meals all the time, and what they ate was based on what was available. With that being said, it means that our bodies are actually also designed to go for a few hours without eating. It can survive without having three square meals a day. Living the IF Life has many benefits which will be explained down below.

Health Benefits

1. You keep yourself full. Some people think that fasting or dieting for that matter, is equal to starvation. However, when Intermittent Fasting is done, Ghrelin, which is a hormone that signals hunger adjusts to the new way of eating of the body which is why you will not feel hungry.

2. You will have better focus and improved concentration. When fasting, catecholamines, which is another hormone of the body is produced more. Therefore, the end result is that you will be more focused on what you are doing.

3. You will have more energy. Since you will not eat as much, there will be less wavering of blood sugar levels. This means that real energy will be more consistent. Plus, you lessen the risk of getting diabetes. You can also exercise while you are on fast, which will actually boost your body's potential to burn more fats. A growth hormone is increased when you fast, which help burn calories.

4. You burn more fat, which means weight loss. Since you eat less and are taking in fewer calories, your body will turn into

body fat to burn for energy, instead of taking the energy from the food that is otherwise eaten on a regular basis if you are not on Intermittent Fasting. This also means that your body will show more of fits lean muscle mass. On a side note, if you are fasting for about 16 hours, your body is already consuming body fat.

5. You will also be able to benefit from the following:

- Less glucose in the blood and better insulin levels

- Less inflammation

- Protection against diseases such as heart disease, Alzheimer's, and cancers

TYPES OF INTERMITTENT FASTING

Intermittent fasting can be accomplished in a number of ways.

The 5/2 method

In this version, you restrict your calories on two consecutive days of the week. This is the most popular intermittent fasting method.

Pick two days of the week, such as Monday and Tuesday. They must be consecutive days. On these two days, only eat 500-600 calories total.

On the other days, you can follow your regular diet. Be sure to not binge on unhealthy foods.

Alternative approaches that have been studied using the 2-day approach include following a complete fast on 2 non-consecutive days, or a significantly lowered calorie intake on 2 non-consecutive days.

The 16/8 method

In this version, you only eat during a eight-hour period, each day.

Skip breakfast every day.

Eat only during a set 8-hour period, such as between 11 a.m. and 7 p.m. You should keep this time consistent every day. You should base these hours on when you need food for energy, such as when you're at work, and when you exercise. During these hours, you should eat mainly unprocessed, whole foods.

Fast for the other 16 hours. You can drink coffee and diet soda, or chew sugar-free gum during this time.

Eat-stop-eat

In this version, you fast for 24 hours at a time.

Once or twice a week, you don't eat from dinner time to dinner time the next day. You fast for 24 hours straight. You can drink calorie-free beverages during these hours.

You can follow your normal diet the other 5 to 6 days per week. You don't need to count calories or restrict your diet on the non-fasting days, although, you should stick to healthy foods as much as possible.

The warrior diet

This version involves eating one meal per day.

Fast for 20 hours per day. You can eat a few servings of raw fruit and veggies, fresh juice, and protein, if needed.

Eat one large meal at night. You should eat veggies first, followed by protein, and then fat. If you're still hungry, you can eat carbohydrates. You can do this only after consuming those foods in the given order.

Risk factors to consider

As with any change to your diet, you should consider the risk factors. You should also consult your doctor prior to beginning any diet program.

Things to consider

If you're diabetic or hypoglycemic, fasting could be dangerous. If you start to feel faint or your body begins to shake, you need to eat.

People with heart problems should not fast. Fasting can make heart problems worse.
Your age can play a part in how well your body deals with the lack of food. Older adults may function better with an overall decrease in calories than with denying themselves food for extended periods of time.

High-level exercisers need the calories to keep their energy levels up, and performance at its best.

Your profession is also an important consideration. If you have a job that keeps you on your feet or requires a high level of concentration, skipping meals may keep you from doing your job to the best of your abilities.

Potential side effects for anyone who fasts include:

- Fatigue

- Dizziness

- Low energy

- Trouble concentrating

If you decide to follow an intermittent fasting diet, you should drink lots of water. This will help with the loss of hydration you may encounter when eating less food.

With the heightened media attention surrounding intermittent fasting, more evidence is needed to support this type of diet. Though, some studies do show that intermittent fasting results in short-term benefits like weight loss, there are few long-term studies. It's still unclear what this type of periodic eating does to eating behaviors, body composition, metabolic rate, and overall health in the long run. It also hasn't been confirmed that intermittent fasting has any advantages over regular daily calorie restriction.

Discuss any question you have with your doctor, and follow their recommendations. You should consider your health history, such as:

- Any issues you've faced with regulating your blood sugar levels

- The impact of fasting on your emotional and psychological state

- Your age

- Your daily activity level before starting this type of diet

- Your Current Weight

PROS AND CONS OF INTERMITTENT-FASTING-DIETS

Intermittent fasting is basically a diet protocol which requires individuals to go through prolonged periods of fasting, in which they will eat virtually nothing (making sure to drink plenty of water) and then, breaking their fasts during certain windows which permit the individual to eat. Some people will fast a few days per week, some people will fast for several hours each day, and some may even go to further extremes. Intermittent fasting has been proven to work, but it is not without it's drawbacks. To help you decide whether or not it could be right for you, we'll now be taking a look at several pros and cons associated with intermittent fasting.

PROS

To begin with, we'll start on a light note, and will look at the positive aspects associated with intermittent fasting diet protocols. Remember, these aren't just opinions, these are hard scientific facts, backed up by years upon years of research and data carried out by the absolute best people in their respective fields.

IT CAN ALTER YOUR HORMONES IN A GOOD WAY

First off, one of the main reasons why intermittent fasting is so popular, not only with people looking to lose weight, but also with bodybuilders as well, is the fact that it has been proven to alter your hormones in a beneficial way internally. When you go through periods of fasting, your insulin levels will drop, which in turn, will facilitate the metabolism of body fat. On top of that, HGH, or Human Growth Hormone levels, can also increase exponentially, by as much as 500% in fact. HGH has been proven to enhance muscle recovery, it enhances muscle growth, and it can even speed up fat loss. Your cells will also repair themselves and function more efficiently for a while. All of these hormonal changes will greatly benefit you; so when the time comes to eat and put some nutrients in your body, you will really be firing on all cylinders, and would have created the perfect anabolic environment for optimal hypertrophy and fat loss.

LOSE FAT

Primarily, this is the biggest reason why people follow intermittent fasting diet plans, and for a very good reason as well. If you're struggling to lose weight, whether you need a little off, or a lot off, intermittent fasting is ideal. You see, the premise is simple: you eat less, and therefore, consume less calories. Ordinarily, you would eat, say, five times per day, including snacks, and often more than that; but with intermittent fasting, as you only eat at certain times, I.E between 5pm and 8pm each night, unless you go on an all-out binge, (which you should not do) you couldn't possibly consume the equivalent of five meals and snacks in calories. As well as consuming fewer calories, your reduced insulin levels and increased HGH levels will also help to facilitate fat loss and speed up the metabolism; so you'll be shedding those pounds in no time at all.

BENEFICIAL FOR THE BODY

As well as providing aesthetical benefits for the body, intermittent fasting has also been found to provide health benefits for the body, on an internal level. Studies have found that intermittent fasting can help to reduce oxidative stress and inflammation within the body, which is hugely beneficial. Oxidative stress, for example, can attack healthy cells and damage them, and potentially cause them to mutate into cancerous cells. Inflammation, as well as being responsible for chronic pain, is also responsible for a number of other very serious ailments, including hypertension, cardiovascular disease, stroke, and heart attack. Intermittent fasting, however, increases the body's immunity to the effects of oxidative stress and inflammation, helping to promote overall health and well-being.

GREAT FOR THE BRAIN

Finally, the last benefit associated with IF which we'll be covering in this article, is the fact that IF is incredibly beneficial for the brain. Numerous metabolic processes within the body will be enhances via IF, many of which provide benefits to the brain as a result. Studies have found that new nerve cells will grow more effectively as a result of IF, plus, they have also revealed that a hormone known as BNDF, or, brain-derived neurotropic factor, will also increase in a fasted environment, and it just so happens that this hormone is also very, very beneficial for the human brain.

CONS

Now that we've looked at the good, let's now look at the not so good, as we look at the cons associated with intermittent fasting. The people who choose the more extreme forms of IF are the most at risk for these possible side effects.

CAN CREATE AN UNHEALTHY RELATIONSHIP WITH FOOD

When it comes to eating disorders and weight loss in general, it is our psychological relationship with food that often plays a key role in what happens next. When you fast, you will be hungry, and if you're at work, or around people eating food, it will look and smell very appealing to you; so from that point onwards, all you will be thinking about is food, how hungry you are, and how long until you get to eat next. This means that your work will suffer, or whatever else it is that you are doing will also suffer because mentally, your judgment and thought processes will be clouded by thoughts of hunger, and what you are going to eat when you break your fast. Overtime, this can create an unhealthy relationship with food which is not what anybody wants.

YOU MAY FEEL SICK WITH HUNGER AT THE BEGINNING

There's no way around it; if you are serious about IF, you must be willing to go through periods of extreme, and by extreme, we mean extreme hunger, numerous times, each week. Being hungry sucks, and we've all heard the jokes about being 'Hangry' (angry with hunger) but for some people, that is true. It can make you irritable, it can affect your relationships, it can affect your concentration levels, and you will feel pretty awful, especially if you are new to IF. If you're mentally strong and know you can deal with these side effects, then great; but if not, you may wish to simply try clean eating and more physical activity.

YOU MAY RELY ON STIMS

When hungry, you have no energy, you feel weak, and you struggle to function. This is why you feel so tired when you wake up in the morning. To counter this, many people drink coffee or other stimulants, which, occasionally are okay, but if you rely on them, this can cause all kinds of risks and dangers to your health. Many IF diet plans allow followers to consume caffeine, usually in the form of black coffee, but the problem is that, the better it makes you feel, the more your body will rely on it when you are feeling tired and weak, and this could lead to addiction. Not only that, caffeine also causes insomnia, upset stomach, and other unpleasant side effects, especially in high dosages.

CORTISOL LEVELS COULD INCREASE

Though the jury is still out on this one, there is evidence which suggests that IF diet plans could elevate cortisol levels, which is the last thing you want. Cortisol is a stress hormone that is responsible for a suppression of the metabolism, for the formation of spots and blemishes, for a drop in beneficial hormones such as HGH, plus it can cause trouble sleeping. When you miss meals, cortisol levels can increase, and metabolism levels can drop, meaning that you will have less energy, and you will also find it much tougher to lose weight as well, which obviously defeats the purpose of the diet in the first place.

POSSIBLE LOSS OF WATER WEIGHT AND MUSCLE

One of the first side effects of fasting is the loss of water and muscle tissue. Because your body isn't being properly hydrated during a fast, your body begins to lose much of it's water weight. This creates a false sense of weight loss for those fasting to lose weight. This is quickly met with disappointment when the pounds easily reappear upon completion of the fast. The significant cut in calories, along with the lack of hydration, leads to a loss of muscle tissue. Loosing muscle makes your body inefficient at fat-burning.

POSSIBLE MALNOURISHMENT

Because you're depriving your body of food and calories, your body will have no source for the nutrients and vitamins it needs to be healthy. This vitamin and nutrient deficiency could result in lowered blood pressure, dry mouth, dizziness and nausea.

POTENTIAL LOWER METABOLISM AND ENERGY

Due to the insufficient amount of calories coming into your body, your system goes into survival mode if you fast for too long. Therefore, your body will work hard to preserve the fat and calories it has stored. While in survival mode, your body lowers your metabolism, causing a decrease in energy levels. This decrease in energy will leave you tired and even stressed. As a result, your work, social life and relationships may be affected.

GET MEDICAL ADVICE

If you are diagnosed with a medical condition that requires consistent medical care, you will need to seek your doctor's professional advice before taking part in any fast. A fast of any kind can alter the effects of prescription medication, and will require close monitoring by a health care professional.

Now let's learn about how to do it right!

INTERMITTENT FASTING FOR BEGINNERS

Intermittent fasting for beginners has two rules to follow:

First: Fasting has to be pleasurable and NOT stressful.

Second: Fasting has to be simple and NOT rigid.

There are two major reasons for people who want to do intermittent fasting (IF) - weight loss or health or both. In any case, it's good to observe these two formulas:

More rules = more complicated = low chance of success

Less rules = less complicated = high chance of success

In terms of health, a 24 hour period off of eating is very healthful; it helps you reduce calories without sacrificing what you like to eat on your non-fasting days, and maybe, even more importantly, it stimulates your body to produce more growth hormone. Yes, that's right, growth hormone; the same one you hear about the celebrities taking to 'stay young.' Growth hormone has many anti-aging benefits, and one of the most interesting being fat burning!

How to do Intermittent Fasting?

In an ideal situation, 2 sessions of 24-hour fast in a week will be good enough to produce significant health and weight loss benefits. However, for beginners, you are not recommended to jump start with a 24-hour fast, unless you are absolutely sure that you can do it.

There is no standard rule of doing IF. Simply try it, and make it work for you. Let simplicity and flexibility be your fasting motto. Don't make it stressful for yourself.

As a beginner to practice intermittent fasting, I would say 'clear your mind from any other weight loss methods, and focus on IF'. This is your first step towards IF success. Think how many times you've been told that breakfast is the most important meal in a day, or you need to eat 6 to 10 small meals a day in order to lose weight. I'm not saying these rules are wrong. If these rules work for you, stay with them. But if you are setting your feets onto the route of intermittent fasting, better put these concepts aside, at least for the period you are trying out IF.

Having your IF mindset ready? Then begin with 'skip meal' and see how your body responds. This is the simplest and easiest way to begin your intermittent fasting journey.

Pick a day to try 'skip breakfast'. Have fresh juice, water or tea instead. No coffee please, unless it's black. If that works out fine, try 'skip lunch' and move on progressively. A 24-hour fast can be done by anybody with an appropriate fasting mindset. One useful tip is not to think of food. Avoid social talk at the pantry over lunch hour. Go out for a walk, or do some simple exercises.

You can also explore these IF options:

- Condensed eating window, e.g. eat ONLY between 11am and 5pm;

- Skip meal on an unplanned basis, as far as it is natural and doesn't interfere in your daily work;

- Early and late, i.e. skip lunch;

- One meal a day, ideally, dinner only when you are relaxed and really have time to enjoy food.

To repeat, fasting has to be pleasurable and not stressful. Don't press hard on yourself. Be flexible. This is very important. Don't upset your boss when you are called upon a business lunch by telling him that you are fasting. Do it as you see fit, and your schedule permits.

Intermittent fasting is a simple long term weight control solution.

SECRETS TO SUCCESSFUL FASTING - FIVE KEYS

Fasting is becoming more and more popular, both as a weight-loss diet, and as a long-term healthy lifestyle choice. Many people have questions about how to set up a fasting diet. Here are five key points to get you started.

1: Choose how long your fast will be

The possibilities here are endless. However, most effective plans use a technique called intermittent fasting. This involves alternating periods of fasting and periods of normal (although healthy) eating. Perhaps, the two most common methods are a 16 hour daily fast (think overnight until lunch the next day), and a 24 hour period one or two times a week. The beauty of both of these schemes is that, they can be made to fit in with you and your life.

2: Drink more water

This is a simple trick that serves two purposes. Firstly, this will increase satiety (the feeling of being full), which is psychologically very important when you are not eating. Secondly, this will accelerate the cleansing effect of a fast, and allow your body to function optimally.

3: Break your fast with a healthy meal

Again, the interest here is twofold. Firstly, when you are getting a healthy meal in first, you are simply leaving less space to eat crap during the rest of your eating "window," which is a guaranteed method to reduce that waistline. Secondly, eating a high sugar meal immediately after fasting will drive your insulin sky-high. Spending your eating hours crashed out in a carb-induced sleep is not the best way to eat! There is one exception here. Does your first meal coincide with training? It is good to release insulin. This will help the body drive nutrients into the muscles, rather than stocking them as fat.

4: Workout regularly

This should be a no-brainer, but working out and particularly weight-training should be at the heart of every diet. This gives you the opportunity to eat more while still burning fat, increases muscle-mass which in turn, increases metabolic rate (meaning, you burn more calories doing nothing) and will make the biggest difference to your appearance in the shortest time.

5: Follow a plan

Again, this should be fairly obvious, but the easiest way to succeed with a diet and exercise regime is to remove any choice. Don't over-think things. By following a plan, you are relying on an expert who has already thought it through. Just follow the instructions.

BONUS: THE SIXTH KEY

If you are really serious about losing weight then add in a workout routine like the one outlined below. Exercise will help speed up fat loss and can also curb hunger.

WEIGHT TRAINING ROUTINE

Weight training is a full body 3 day routine. Again, exact days don't really matter, but make sure you have a day off in between workouts. You will be working the large muscles only (legs, back, chest) on days 1 and 2, and will add in the smaller muscles arms/calves) on day 3. You will do 4 sets of 6-8 reps for each large muscle, and 2-3 sets of 8-12 for the smaller ones.

Here is a sample workout routine:

Day 1: Push
Flat Bench Press / Shoulder Press / Leg Press / Weighted Crunches

Day 2: Pull
Rows / Chinups / Hamstring Curl

Day 3: Push/Pull
Incline Bench Press / Rows / Squats / Calf Raises / Lateral Raise / Barbell Curl / Tricep Pushdown / Lateral Raise / Back Extensions / Weighted Crunches

For maximum fat loss, cardio should be down 2-3 times per week. Start with a 5 minute warm up, and then begin 10 minutes of High Intensity Interval Training, or HIIT. This works best on an elliptical or a spin bike, instead of a treadmill. You will do this in 1 minute intervals. Max intensity for 1 minute, followed by a moderate pace for 1 minute. Repeat until 10 minutes are up. After the HIIT session is over, drink some water and rest for 5 minutes. After your rest, do 30 minutes of Low to Moderate Intensity, Steady State Cardio. A treadmill works great for this. Don't forget to wait an hour and have your 50g of protein.

POPULAR WAYS TO DO INTERMITTENT FASTING

Intermittent fasting has been very trendy in recent years.

It is claimed to cause weight loss, improve metabolic health and perhaps, even extend lifespan.

Not surprisingly given the popularity, several different types/ methods of intermittent fasting have been devised.

All of them can be effective, but which one fits best will depend on the individual.

Here are popular ways to do intermittent fasting.

1. The 16/8 Method: Fast for 16 hours each day.

The 16/8 Method involves fasting every day for 14-16 hours, and restricting your daily "eating window" to 8-10 hours.

Within the eating window, you can fit in 2, 3 or more meals.

Doing this method of fasting can actually be as simple as not eating anything after dinner, and skipping breakfast.

For example, if you finish your last meal at 8 pm, and then don't eat until 12 noon the next day, then you are technically fasting for 16 hours between meals.

It is generally recommended that women only fast 14-15 hours, because they seem to do better with slightly shorter fasts.

For people who get hungry in the morning and like to eat breakfast, then this can be hard to get used to at first. However, many breakfast skippers actually instinctively eat this way.

You can drink water, coffee and other non-caloric beverages during the fast, and this can help reduce hunger levels.

It is very important to eat mostly healthy foods during your eating window. This won't work if you eat lots of junk food, or excessive amounts of calories.

Bottom Line: The 16/8 method involves daily fasts of 16 hours for men, and 14-15 hours for women. On each day, you restrict your eating to an 8-10 hour "eating window" where you can fit in 2-3 or more meals.

2. The 5:2 Diet: Fast for 2 days per week.

The 5:2 diet involves eating normally 5 days of the week, while restricting calories to 500-600 on two days of the week.

This diet is also called the Fast diet, and was popularized by British journalist, and doctor Michael Mosley.

On the fasting days, it is recommended that women eat 500 calories, and men 600 calories.

For example, you might eat normally on all days except Mondays and Thursdays, where you eat two small meals (250 calories per meal for women, and 300 for men).

As critics correctly point out, there are no studies testing the 5:2 diet itself, but there are plenty of studies on the benefits of intermittent fasting.

Bottom Line: The 5:2 diet, or the Fast diet, involves eating 500-600 calories for two days of the week, but eating normally the other 5 days.

3. Eat-Stop-Eat: Do a 24-hour fast, once or twice a week.

Eat-Stop-Eat involves a 24-hour fast, either once or twice per week.

By fasting from dinner one day, to dinner the next, this amounts to a 24-hour fast.

For example, if you finish dinner on Monday at 7 pm, and don't eat until dinner the next day at 7 pm, then you've just done a full 24-hour fast.

You can also fast from breakfast to breakfast, or lunch to lunch. The end result is the same. Water, coffee and other non-caloric beverages are allowed during the fast, but no solid food.

If you are doing this to lose weight, then it is very important that you eat normally during the eating periods. As in, eat the same amount of food as if you hadn't been fasting at all.

The problem with this method is that a full 24-hour fast can be fairly difficult for many people.

However, you don't need to go all-in right away, starting with 14-16 hours and then moving upwards from there is fine.

Bottom Line: Eat-Stop-Eat is an intermittent fasting program with one or two 24-hour fasts per week.

4. Alternate-Day Fasting: Fast every other day.

Alternate-Day fasting means fasting every other day.

There are several different versions of this. Some of them allow about 500 calories during the fasting days.

Many of the lab studies showing health benefits of intermittent fasting used some version of this.

A full fast every other day seems rather extreme; so I do not recommend this for beginners.

With this method, you will be going to bed very hungry several times per week, which is not very pleasant, and probably unsustainable in the long-term.

Bottom Line: Alternate-day fasting means fasting every other day, either by not eating anything, or only eating a few hundred calories.

5. The Warrior Diet: Fast during the day, eat a huge meal at night.

It involves eating small amounts of raw fruits and vegetables during the day, then eating one huge meal at night.

Basically, you "fast" all day and "feast" at night within a 4 hour eating window.

The Warrior Diet was one of the first popular "diets" to include a form of intermittent fasting.

This diet also emphasizes food choices that are quite similar to a paleo diet – whole, unprocessed foods that resemble what they looked like in nature.

Bottom Line: The Warrior Diet is about eating only small amounts of vegetables and fruits during the day, then eating one huge meal at night.

6. Spontaneous Meal Skipping: Skip meals when convenient.

You don't actually need to follow a structured intermittent fasting plan to reap some of the benefits.

Another option is to simply skip meals from time to time, when you don't feel hungry or are too busy to cook and eat.

It is a myth that people need to eat every few hours, or they will hit "starvation mode" or lose muscle.

The human body is well equipped to handle long periods of famine, let alone, missing one or two meals from time to time.

So if you're really not hungry one day, skip breakfast and just eat a healthy lunch and dinner. Or if you're travelling somewhere and can't find anything you want to eat, do a short fast.

Skipping 1 or 2 meals when you feel so inclined is basically a spontaneous intermittent fast. Just make sure to eat healthy foods at the other meals.

Bottom Line: Another more "natural" way to do intermittent fasting is to simply skip 1 or 2 meals when you don't feel hungry or don't have time to eat.

A DEEPER LOOK AT THE PROTOCOLS

The benefits of IF varies from hormonal management to caloric reduction and decreased hunger, and which benefits are prioritized will be dependent on which "type" of IF you use.

This ebook will give you a complete analysis of the most popular intermittent fasting styles currently discussed in the fitness world, benefits and drawbacks, as well as my own personal experience.

Given that the most obvious difference between each of these methods is the length of the fasting period; below, you will find each listed from longest fast to shortest.

24-Hour Fast (aka Eat-Stop-Eat)

SUMMARY: A 24-hour fasting period is essentially what it sounds like: if your last meal is at 8pm on Monday, then you simply do not eat again (at all) until Tuesday at 8pm. This can be done 1-3 times per week, with 2 being the most common iteration.

BENEFITS: The 24-hour fast works well for a number of reasons. The first of these is that it is easily adaptable to any lifestyle, and it's very hard to screw up. The only rule is "don't eat" for 24 hours. As mentioned above, this is much easier than a 36 hour fast, especially for those new to it.

Secondly, like most methods of fasting, the abstinence from caloric intake for large periods of time is going to be a large part of the reason for success.
For example, if you generally eat 2,000 calories every day, that's 14,000 calories over the course of a week.

If you remove two of those days, you're eating 4,000 calories less. Without any other changes to your lifestyle, you'd be on pace for over a pound of fat per week. Even if you "compensate" and eat a little more on the days you're not fasting, you are still going to wind up with a fairly substantial caloric deficit. Add in some exercise, and it's not hard to see consistent weight loss.

Caloric manipulation aside, this style of fasting works incredibly well because of the effect that fasting has on your overall hormonal environment.

More specifically, when we talk about fasting, we're really going to talk about two hormones: insulin and growth hormone.

With regard to insulin, it seems that the less often you eat, the less often you raise insulin levels. This is not surprising, obviously. It's even less surprising that this would lead to fat loss, since we know that chronically elevated insulin levels make it very difficult to lose fat.

Therefore, if you're eating less often, you're going to have less insulin issues—even if you're eating the same foods in the same amounts. (This, by way, is a pretty strong argument against the popular frequent feeding method of 5-6 meals per day). However, while fasting, infrequent feeding helps to control insulin and keep it low, that's not enough to stimulate fat loss...unless growth hormone is present.

That is, if insulin AND growth hormone are both low, there isn't a huge effect on fat loss. And so, while insulin management is important, growth hormone management is even more important.

Which brings us to the very predictable point: The effect of fasting on growth hormone is incredibly important.

Your body releases GH pretty consistently, but research has shown increased secretion of growth hormone in three specific instances:

- During or immediately after sleep

- After exercise (as little as 10 minutes)

- During and immediately after a fast

Looking at these three things—all of which are thoroughly discussed in Pilon's Eat-Stop-Eat—it's not hard to come up with a "best of all worlds" scenario.

If you produce a lot of GH while sleeping, and you produce it while fasting, then the obvious way to combine these is to continue fasting after you wake, allowing for prolonged GH secretion; from there, exercise will allow for increased production in addition to your prolonged secretion.

Overall, this maximizes both the presence of GH and it's effect; and in addition, the elevated GH in combination with the low insulin is a deadly one-two punch to your body fat.

Finally, one of the main benefits of both this style of fasting and the book itself is the incredible flexibility of the program, and the ease with which you can adapt it to your lifestyle—you can fast any day you like, and can move it around at will to suit your social life, which is important.

DRAWBACKS: There aren't many here. The main problem that clients of mine seem to have here is that 24 hours seems like a long time to go without food; however, this is not unique to 24-hour fasting.

That said, there are some people who seem to have genuine problems with abstaining from food for significant length of time—in particular, people with low blood sugar seem to have an issue with it. If you fall into this category, you may want to tread lightly.

The only other real problem here would be for people who don't want to miss out on post-workout nutrition, but find the need to train on fast days. This can be alleviated by either moving your workout to the end of the fasting period, or simply scheduling your off days and fast days to coincide.

20-Hour Fast (aka Warrior Diet)

SUMMARY: Simply, the diet is, in theory, a 20-hour fast followed by a 4-hour feeding period; as the name implies, this is inspired by the nutritional habits of the warriors of antiquity, who certainly weren't in the habit of eating six meals per day.

Instead, warriors in cultures, ranging from Roman centurions to the Spartan elite, subsisted on one to two meals: a large meal in the evening and (sometimes), a small meal in the morning; according to the author that is.

The diet itself is modeled after this type of eating schedule; however, it's worth noting that this is often criticized for not being "true" in IF.

That is, in most cases, while having a small breakfast and a large dinner will probably work for weight loss, there may only be 8-10 hours between them...which, some people posit, isn't long enough to get the benefits of fasting.

Moreover, during the fasting part of the day, the diet allows for mild consumption—you'd be allowed to eat a few servings of raw fruits and vegetables, and a few servings of protein (protein shakes included) if needed/wanted. These are kept quite small. Having said that, some fasting purists understandably maintain that Warrior Dieting, should you choose to exercise these options, is not fasting.

In practice, however, most people skip the small meal, and simply have one large meal at the end of the day.

BENEFITS: Much like a 24-hour fast, a 20-hour fast allows you to reap the hormonal benefit of increased growth hormone. And, like all fasting, will generally result in fewer calories being consumed.

The benefit that is unique to this type of fasting is that you're generally eating one large meal and, therefore, the make up of such a meal isn't as important as you might think; as long as you get adequate protein, you can eat "junkier" foods and still do well.
Moreover, having only one meal makes life pretty simple, and less thinking means less screw-ups.

DRAWBACKS: On the flip side of that coin, once again, we're running into the issue of hunger; and again, this isn't unique to Warrior Dieting.

The main drawback in my experience comes from the meal itself—trying to get all of your calories in a single meal means that meal is, by necessity, quite large; so large, in fact, that eating it often leads to discomfort. This is why many people turn to less wholesome foods: getting in 2000 calories of chicken, veggies and rice isn't nearly as easy as getting it in chicken wings and French fries.

16/8 Fasting (aka LeanGains)

SUMMARY: Popularized by Martin Berkhan, LeanGains or 16/8 is a style of IF where the fasting period is 16 hours, and the feeding window is shortened to 8 hours; during this time, users may eat as few meals as they like, with the most frequent iteration being three meals.

Designed specifically with training in mind, and mean to to be used for such, the 16/8 method has specific post-workout suggestions and recommendations, and, in nearly all ways, is the most sophisticated form of intermittent fasting.

BENEFITS: In addition to having all of the benefits inherent in other types of fasting, the 16/8 methods is a stand out because it offers an advanced level of hormonal management.

While something like 24-Hour fasting or Alternate Day Fasting will give you these benefits, these methods are not for daily practice, whereas 16/8 is. This means that you are going to have a daily increase in GH, which leads to greater effects.

Moreover, daily practice (obviously) means that you're eating the same way every day; this means that you don't experience ups and downs in hunger, as with some other forms of fasting. (Put another way, some people experience difficulty with fasting for 24-36 hours because they do it infrequently; not an issue with daily practice).

Going from there, there is also the benefit of hunger management. A number of studies have recently shown that larger, infrequent meals are better for satiety than small, frequent meals—so you'll be fuller, longer.

DRAWBACKS: There are very few drawbacks to this style of IF, and these mainly come from scheduling. You see, from everything seen and read, the LG protocol is MOST effective if the workout is performed in a fasted state, and the meal that breaks the fast is immediately post workouts.

For some, execution can become a little impractical; for most people, adhering to that simple rule forces them to shift the feeding window to inconvenient times.

Given that we want to have a 16-hour fasting window that ends with the PWO meal, and begin an 8-hour feeding window, you can see how either of those times present some issues. For example, let's look at 6am. In order for this to work as your first meal, your last meal is going to be at 4pm (allowing you to fast for 16 hours for your next feeding window).

Right off the bat, see three (theoretical) problems arising here.

This first is that having your last meal at 4pm can present some social issues, at least if you ever want to have dinner with your friends or family. (The exception is Sunday "dinner" in any Italian household, which for some reason, inexplicably begins around noon and ends just after sundown.)

The second is that your feeding window is going to coincide almost minute for minute with your workday, making it difficult to eat your meals, let alone enjoy them.

The third problem is that a good number of your fasting hours are after your feeding hours have ended. That said, if you're looking to try 16/8, and can only work out in the AM, it's certainly doable; just be aware of this going in. And, of course, this "problem" is really only applicable to certain people.

Like any other style of eating, make it work for you—within the rules of the system.
Of all intermittent fasting protocols, 16/8 is probably the most sophisticated, in terms of both intention and execution. While most fasting is effective mainly because it prevents you from eating, the LeanGains style is really about taking control your hormones. Which is awesome.

This style of IF is best for serious folks, and those who are already lean; and, again, this is the ONLY style of IF that was designed specifically with fitness-oriented people in mind, and therefore, yields exceptional results for folks who train consistently.

INTERMITTENT FASTING PROTOCOLS WRAP UP

That's about it! You now have a very firm overview of the most popular types of Intermittent Fasting, as well as the benefits and drawbacks of each. If you're looking to try an IF plan, simply choose from those above, and read up on them.

While all of them are effective, the most important thing is to choose the one that fits in best with your lifestyle, and give yourself the greatest advantage.

One final point: specifically because IF is not a diet, it lends itself well to nearly anything that is a diet. That means that you can practice intermittent fasting regardless of your nutritional restrictions or preferences—it doesn't matter if you're a low carb-er, a Paleo dieter, lactose free, vegan, or anything in between; you can simply apply the IF system of your choice to your current diet.

This is because, intermittent fasting is a way of eating a nutritional lifestyle that will allow you to reach your goals in an efficient and convenient manner, and then, hold onto your physique when you achieve them.

INTERMITTENT FASTING FOR WOMEN

For women who are interested in weight loss, intermittent fasting may seem like a great choice, but many people want to know; should women fast? Is intermittent fasting effective for women? There have been a few key studies about intermittent fasting which can help to shed some light on this interesting new dietary trend.

Intermittent fasting is also known as alternate-day fasting, although there are certainly some variations on this diet. The American Journal of Clinical Nutrition performed a study recently, that enrolled 16 obese men and women on a 10-week program. On the fasting days, participants consumed food to 25% of their estimated energy needs. The rest of the time, they received dietary counseling, but were not given a specific guideline to follow during this time.

As expected, the participants lost weight due to this study, but what researchers really found interesting were some specific changes. The subjects were all still obese after just 10 weeks, but they had shown improvement in cholesterol, LDL-cholesterol, triglycerides, and systolic blood pressure. What made this an interesting find was that most people have to lose more weight than these study participants before seeing the same changes. It was a fascinating find which has spurred a great number of people to try fasting.

Intermittent fasting for women has some beneficial effects. What makes it especially important for women who are trying to lose weight is that women have a much higher fat proportion in their bodies. When trying to lose weight, the body primarily burns through carbohydrate stores with the first 6 hours, and then starts to burn fat. Women who are following a healthy diet and exercise plan may be struggling with stubborn fat, but fasting is a realistic solution to this.

Intermittent Fasting For Women Over 50

Obviously, our bodies and our metabolism changes when we hit menopause. One of the biggest changes that women over 50 experience is that they have a slower metabolism, and they start to put on weight. Fasting may be a good way to reverse and prevent this weight gain though. Studies have shown that this fasting pattern helps to regulate appetite, and people who follow it regularly do not experience the same cravings that others do. If you're over 50 and trying to adjust to your slower metabolism, intermittent fasting can help you to avoid eating too much on a daily basis.

When you reach 50, your body also starts to develop some chronic diseases like high cholesterol, and high blood pressure. Intermittent fasting has been shown to decrease both cholesterol and blood pressure, even without a great deal of weight loss. If you've started to notice your numbers rising at the doctor's office each year, you may be able to bring them back down with fasting, even without losing much weight.

Intermittent fasting may not be a great idea for every woman. Anyone with a specific health condition or who tends to be hypoglycemic should consult a doctor. However, this new dietary trend has specific benefits for women who naturally store more fat in their bodies, and may have trouble getting rid of these fat stores.

Is IF good for women?

Before listing intermittent fasting pros and cons for women, first realize there is no single definition of Intermittent Fasting. Various (and confusing) versions of IF might include:

Don't eat between 7 PM and 7 AM

Only eat during a 6 or 8 hour window, such as 12 PM to 7 PM

Just skip breakfast

Reduce calories by only eating twice daily (calorie restriction)

Eat all you want in the hours allotted (no calorie restriction)

Fast anytime you want.

  Once weekly. Three times weekly. Off and on for several months.

Oh, and there's a 7th option: drink coffee with butter and MCT oil as breakfast, but no other breakfast.   This is called Bulletproof Intermittent Fasting.

Another version of all this gets into Ketogenic Diets, where fat is a major source of calories, and proteins and carbs are reduced. Many people assume IF and Keto go together, but they are different diets with different goals, and yes, some people do them together.

MORE REASONS TO TRY INTERMITTENT FASTING

So, you want to lose weight, and you have chosen to lose weight by intermittent fasting. For those of you who don't know, intermittent fasting is simply a system that alternates between periods of eating and not eating (usually, you get to consume water and sometimes, low-calorie drinks such as black coffee)

What this means is that for a set time, you get to eat and then, you cut down on the amount of calories you take in.

Pretty cool right? That is like a very wonderful idea. I get to eat whatever I want for some time. Later, I cut down on the intake of calories. And the best news is that I get to lose weight.

Intermittent fasting has been around for a while, and research has shown that it comes with a lot of health benefits.

Getting really interesting? Apart from losing weight, it also comes with a lot of health benefits.

It reduces your urge to get hungry while dieting. For someone looking to start dieting, you definitely know that controlling that hunger urge is a massive work to accomplish. But after a few days of starting the Intermittent fasting, your body adjusts to this new eating pattern.

It increases your mental focus and concentration. As you are fasting, your body releases a chemical called catecholamine, which significantly increases your mental awareness, and your productivity.

It stabilizes your energy levels, and improves your mood. With fewer meals, your blood sugar levels will be kept stable. This will lead to constant energy levels, and help you avoid diabetes in the long run.

Reduced oxidative stress. This simply means that as you fast, it reduces the accumulation of oxidative radicals in the body. This will greatly reduce damage to harm caused to internal organs in your body.

It increases your capacity to resist stress, disease and aging. Intermittent fasting, just like exercising, induces a cellular stress response in your body, which increases your capacity to cope with stress, and resist disease and aging.

You get to burn fat. Obviously this is the main reason. You get to lose excess weight. When you eat, your body uses up the glycogen from the food you just ate to give you energy. But as you fast, your body switches to the stored fats, and uses them for energy.
It saves you time and money. Eating fewer meals means preparing and buying fewer meals. Hence, you save money and time. Also, you are less exposed to flavors and are therefore, less likely to get bored and eat something you should not.

CONCLUSION

There are a lot of people getting great results with some of these methods.

That being said, if you're already happy with your health, and don't see much room for improvement, then feel free to safely ignore all of this.

Intermittent fasting is not for everyone. It is not something that anyone needs to do; it is just another tool in the toolbox that can be useful for some people.

Some also believe that it may not be as beneficial for women as men, and it may also be a poor choice for people who are prone to eating disorders.

If you decide to try this out, then keep in mind that you need to eat healthy as well.

It is not possible to binge on junk foods during the eating periods, and expect to lose weight and improve health. Calories still count, and food quality is still absolutely crucial.

But at the end of the day, what really needs to be said is congratulations! Congratulations on making the decision to buy this book and start taking steps towards achieving your long term health goals!

NOTE FROM THE AUTHOR

You have my sincere thanks for buying this book! If you feel like you got some value from this book please share that with others. Leave my book an Amazon review, reviews really help.

Thanks so much,

Eden